# THE COMPLETE HEART HEALTHY COOKBOOK FOR DIABETICS

## Boost Heart Health and Manage Diabetes with the Ultimate Cookbook

**Dr Lily Morgan**

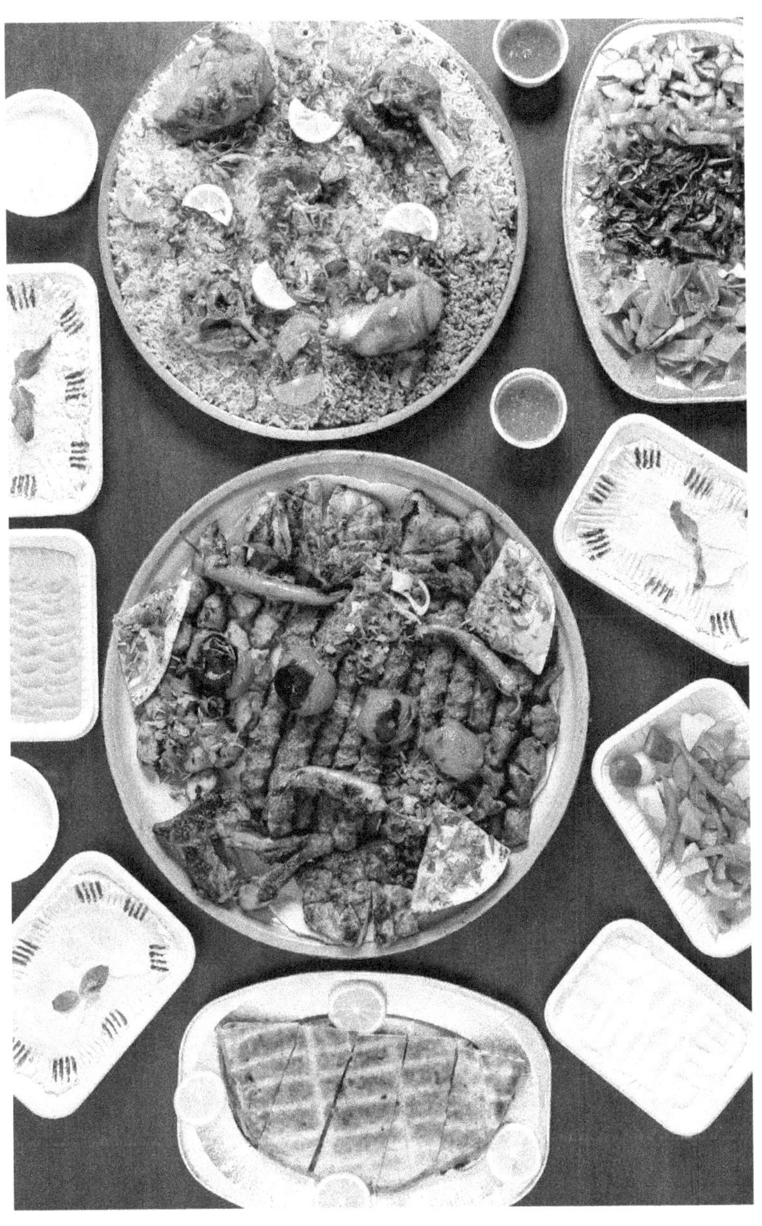

# TABLE OF CONTENTS

## Chapter 6: Desserts ...................................................90

# INTRODUCTION

In the vast realm of culinary delights, the convergence of heart-healthy cooking and diabetes management has emerged as a crucial topic of interest. The journey towards maintaining a healthy heart while effectively managing diabetes can be daunting, but with the right knowledge, skills, and recipes at hand, it becomes an empowering and fulfilling endeavor. This chapter serves as the gateway to the world of "The Complete Heart Healthy Cookbook for Diabetics," offering a comprehensive introduction that will lay the foundation for your culinary adventure.

## Understanding Heart-Healthy Diabetic Cooking

To embark on this journey, it is essential to grasp the essence of heart-healthy diabetic cooking. This section delves into the core principles that guide this culinary approach, exploring the intricate relationship between diabetes and heart health. You will gain insights into the importance of maintaining balanced blood sugar levels, managing cholesterol and blood pressure, and adopting a nutrient-rich diet that nourishes both your heart and body.

## Importance of Nutrition for Heart Health and Diabetes Management

Nutrition serves as the cornerstone of both heart health and diabetes management. In this section, we delve into the significance of proper nutrition in promoting a healthy heart and effectively managing diabetes. Discover the role of essential nutrients, such as fiber, healthy fats, lean proteins, and complex carbohydrates, in supporting cardiovascular well-being while keeping blood sugar levels stable. Uncover the power of mindful eating, portion control, and creating a well-balanced plate to optimize your health.

## Guidelines for a Heart-Healthy Diabetic Diet

Navigating the vast array of dietary recommendations can be overwhelming, especially when you are striving for a heart-healthy diabetic diet. This section presents a comprehensive set of guidelines tailored specifically for individuals with diabetes who are looking to prioritize their heart health. From understanding the importance of carbohydrates and glycemic index to incorporating a variety of colorful fruits and vegetables, you will gain practical advice on crafting a diet that supports your overall well-being.

## Essential Ingredients and Cooking Techniques

Arming yourself with knowledge about essential ingredients and cooking techniques is crucial when venturing into heart-healthy diabetic cooking. In this section, we explore a range of key ingredients that form the building blocks of nutritious and delicious meals. From whole grains and legumes to lean proteins and heart-friendly fats, you will learn how to select and prepare ingredients that enhance flavor, texture, and nutritional value. Additionally, we will discuss various cooking techniques that help retain the health benefits of your ingredients while ensuring a delightful culinary experience.

# Tips for Meal Planning and Grocery Shopping

Effective meal planning and smart grocery shopping are indispensable skills when embarking on a heart-healthy diabetic journey. This section provides practical tips and strategies to streamline your meal planning process, ensuring you have nourishing and delectable meals throughout the week. You will learn how to create a balanced meal plan, make a comprehensive grocery list, and optimize your shopping experience to ensure you have all the ingredients necessary for your heart-healthy diabetic recipes.

## Kitchen Tools and Equipment

Equipping your kitchen with the right tools and equipment is instrumental in preparing heart-healthy diabetic meals with ease and efficiency. This section explores a range of essential kitchen tools and gadgets that will elevate your culinary prowess. From quality knives and cutting boards to measuring cups and food scales, you will discover the must-have tools that simplify your cooking process and contribute to your success in the kitchen. Additionally, we will touch upon kitchen organization tips to create a functional and inspiring cooking space.

# Chapter 1: 30-Day Meal Plan

Enjoy a variety of delicious and nutritious recipes designed to support heart health and manage diabetes. Feel free to repeat the meal plan or explore more recipes from the cookbook to continue your healthy eating journey.

## Week 1:

**Day 1:**

Breakfast: Hearty Oatmeal with Berries and Nuts

Lunch: Grilled Chicken and Vegetable Salad with Balsamic Vinaigrette

Dinner: Grilled Salmon with Lemon and Dill

Snack: Roasted Red Pepper Hummus with Veggie Sticks

Dessert: Fresh Berry Parfait with Whipped Cream

Smoothie: Green Power Smoothie with Spinach and Kale

**Day 2:**

Breakfast: Vegetable and Egg White Scramble

Lunch: Turkey and Hummus Wrap with Fresh Vegetables

Dinner: Baked Chicken Breast with Herbs and Garlic

Snack: Baked Sweet Potato Chips with Yogurt Dip

Dessert: Chocolate Avocado Mousse

Smoothie: Berry Blast Smoothie with Greek Yogurt

**Day 3:**

Breakfast: Whole Wheat Pancakes with Sugar-Free Syrup

Lunch: Quinoa and Black Bean Salad with Lime Dressing

Dinner: Shrimp and Broccoli Stir-Fry with Brown Rice

Snack: Avocado and Tomato Salsa with Whole Wheat Pita Chips

Dessert: Greek Yogurt and Fruit Popsicles

Smoothie: Tropical Paradise Smoothie with Pineapple and Coconut

**Day 4:**

Breakfast: Greek Yogurt Parfait with Fresh Fruit

Lunch: Salmon and Quinoa Bowl with Lemon-Dill Dressing

Dinner: Turkey Chili with Beans and Veggies

Snack: Greek Yogurt and Berry Popsicles

Dessert: Baked Apple with Cinnamon and Walnuts

Smoothie: Chocolate Peanut Butter Banana Smoothie

**Day 5:**

Breakfast: Spinach and Mushroom Frittata

Lunch: Mediterranean Chickpea Salad with Feta Cheese

Dinner: Spinach and Feta Stuffed Chicken Breast

Snack: Cucumber and Tuna Bites

Dessert: Mixed Berry Crumble with Oat Topping

Smoothie: Spinach and Mango Smoothie with Almond Milk


**Day 6:**

Breakfast: Quinoa Breakfast Bowl with Almonds and Cinnamon

Lunch: Tofu Stir-Fry with Brown Rice

Dinner: Eggplant and Chickpea Curry with Brown Rice

Snack: Spiced Nuts and Seeds Mix

Dessert: Chia Seed Pudding with Berries

Smoothie: Antioxidant-Rich Blueberry Smoothie


**Day 7:**

Breakfast: Smoked Salmon and Avocado Toast

Lunch: Lentil Soup with Spinach and Tomatoes

Dinner: Beef and Vegetable Stir-Fry with Quinoa

Snack: Edamame and Sea Salt

Dessert: Frozen Banana Bites with Dark Chocolate

Smoothie: Peach and Ginger Smoothie with Flaxseed

## Week 2:

**Day 8:**

Breakfast: Blueberry Almond Smoothie Bowl

Lunch: Caprese Salad with Basil Pesto

Dinner: Ratatouille with Herbed Quinoa

Snack: Zucchini Fritters with Greek Yogurt Sauce

Dessert: Lemon Blueberry Bars with Almond Crust

Smoothie: Raspberry and Almond Butter Smoothie

**Day 9:**

Breakfast: Apple Cinnamon Overnight Oats

Lunch: Roasted Vegetable and Quinoa Stuffed Bell Peppers

Dinner: Baked Cod with Tomato and Olive Relish

Snack: Stuffed Mushrooms with Spinach and Cheese

Dessert: Pumpkin Spice Energy Balls

Smoothie: Pineapple and Cucumber Smoothie with Mint

**Day 10:**

Breakfast: Veggie Packed Breakfast Burrito

Lunch: Greek-Style Chicken Wrap with Tzatziki Sauce

Dinner: Vegetarian Enchiladas with Black Beans and Sweet Potato

Snack: Mini Vegetable Quiches

Dessert: Mango and Coconut Rice Pudding

Smoothie: Coffee and Banana Smoothie with Oatmeal

**Day 11:**

Breakfast: Hearty Oatmeal with Berries and Nuts

Lunch: Grilled Chicken and Vegetable Salad with Balsamic Vinaigrette

Dinner: Grilled Salmon with Lemon and Dill

Snack: Roasted Red Pepper Hummus with Veggie Sticks

Dessert: Fresh Berry Parfait with Whipped Cream

Smoothie: Green Power Smoothie with Spinach and Kale

**Day 12:**

Breakfast: Vegetable and Egg White Scramble

Lunch: Turkey and Hummus Wrap with Fresh Vegetables

Dinner: Baked Chicken Breast with Herbs and Garlic

Snack: Baked Sweet Potato Chips with Yogurt Dip

Dessert: Chocolate Avocado Mousse

Smoothie: Berry Blast Smoothie with Greek Yogurt


## Day 13:

Breakfast: Whole Wheat Pancakes with Sugar-Free Syrup

Lunch: Quinoa and Black Bean Salad with Lime Dressing

Dinner: Shrimp and Broccoli Stir-Fry with Brown Rice

Snack: Avocado and Tomato Salsa with Whole Wheat Pita Chips

Dessert: Greek Yogurt and Fruit Popsicles

Smoothie: Tropical Paradise Smoothie with Pineapple and Coconut


## Day 14:

Breakfast: Greek Yogurt Parfait with Fresh Fruit

Lunch: Salmon and Quinoa Bowl with Lemon-Dill Dressing

Dinner: Turkey Chili with Beans and Veggies

Snack: Greek Yogurt and Berry Popsicles

Dessert: Baked Apple with Cinnamon and Walnuts

Smoothie: Chocolate Peanut Butter Banana Smoothie

# Week 3:

**Day 15:**

Breakfast: Spinach and Mushroom Frittata

Lunch: Mediterranean Chickpea Salad with Feta Cheese

Dinner: Spinach and Feta Stuffed Chicken Breast

Snack: Cucumber and Tuna Bites

Dessert: Mixed Berry Crumble with Oat Topping

Smoothie: Spinach and Mango Smoothie with Almond Milk

**Day 16:**

Breakfast: Quinoa Breakfast Bowl with Almonds and Cinnamon

Lunch: Tofu Stir-Fry with Brown Rice

Dinner: Eggplant and Chickpea Curry with Brown Rice

Snack: Spiced Nuts and Seeds Mix

Dessert: Chia Seed Pudding with Berries

Smoothie: Antioxidant-Rich Blueberry Smoothie

**Day 17:**

Breakfast: Smoked Salmon and Avocado Toast

Lunch: Lentil Soup with Spinach and Tomatoes

Dinner: Beef and Vegetable Stir-Fry with Quinoa

Snack: Edamame and Sea Salt

Dessert: Frozen Banana Bites with Dark Chocolate

Smoothie: Peach and Ginger Smoothie with Flaxseed

**Day 18:**

Breakfast: Blueberry Almond Smoothie Bowl

Lunch: Caprese Salad with Basil Pesto

Dinner: Ratatouille with Herbed Quinoa

Snack: Zucchini Fritters with Greek Yogurt Sauce

Dessert: Lemon Blueberry Bars with Almond Crust

Smoothie: Raspberry and Almond Butter Smoothie

**Day 19:**

Breakfast: Apple Cinnamon Overnight Oats

Lunch: Roasted Vegetable and Quinoa Stuffed Bell Peppers

Dinner: Baked Cod with Tomato and Olive Relish

Snack: Stuffed Mushrooms with Spinach and Cheese

Dessert: Pumpkin Spice Energy Balls

Smoothie: Pineapple and Cucumber Smoothie with Mint

**Day 20:**

Breakfast: Veggie Packed Breakfast Burrito

Lunch: Greek-Style Chicken Wrap with Tzatziki Sauce

Dinner: Vegetarian Enchiladas with Black Beans and Sweet Potato

Snack: Mini Vegetable Quiches

Dessert: Mango and Coconut Rice Pudding

Smoothie: Coffee and Banana Smoothie with Oatmeal

**Day 21:**

Breakfast: Hearty Oatmeal with Berries and Nuts

Lunch: Grilled Chicken and Vegetable Salad with Balsamic Vinaigrette

Dinner: Grilled Salmon with Lemon and Dill

Snack: Roasted Red Pepper Hummus with Veggie Sticks

Dessert: Fresh Berry Parfait with Whipped Cream

Smoothie: Green Power Smoothie with Spinach and Kale

## Week 4:

**Day 22:**

Breakfast: Vegetable and Egg White Scramble

Lunch: Turkey and Hummus Wrap with Fresh Vegetables

Dinner: Baked Chicken Breast with Herbs and Garlic

Snack: Baked Sweet Potato Chips with Yogurt Dip

Dessert: Chocolate Avocado Mousse

Smoothie: Berry Blast Smoothie with Greek Yogurt

**Day 23:**

Breakfast: Whole Wheat Pancakes with Sugar-Free Syrup

Lunch: Quinoa and Black Bean Salad with Lime Dressing

Dinner: Shrimp and Broccoli Stir-Fry with Brown Rice

Snack: Avocado and Tomato Salsa with Whole Wheat Pita Chips

Dessert: Greek Yogurt and Fruit Popsicles

Smoothie: Tropical Paradise Smoothie with Pineapple and Coconut

**Day 24:**

Breakfast: Greek Yogurt Parfait with Fresh Fruit

Lunch: Salmon and Quinoa Bowl with Lemon-Dill Dressing

Dinner: Turkey Chili with Beans and Veggies

Snack: Greek Yogurt and Berry Popsicles

Dessert: Baked Apple with Cinnamon and Walnuts

Smoothie: Chocolate Peanut Butter Banana Smoothie

**Day 25:**

Breakfast: Spinach and Mushroom Frittata

Lunch: Mediterranean Chickpea Salad with Feta Cheese

Dinner: Spinach and Feta Stuffed Chicken Breast

Snack: Cucumber and Tuna Bites

Dessert: Mixed Berry Crumble with Oat Topping

Smoothie: Spinach and Mango Smoothie with Almond
Milk

**Day 26:**

Breakfast: Quinoa Breakfast Bowl with Almonds and
Cinnamon

Lunch: Tofu Stir-Fry with Brown Rice

Dinner: Eggplant and Chickpea Curry with Brown Rice

Snack: Spiced Nuts and Seeds Mix

Dessert: Chia Seed Pudding with Berries

Smoothie: Antioxidant-Rich Blueberry Smoothie

**Day 27:**

Breakfast: Smoked Salmon and Avocado Toast

Lunch: Lentil Soup with Spinach and Tomatoes

Dinner: Beef and Vegetable Stir-Fry with Quinoa

Snack: Edamame and Sea Salt

Dessert: Frozen Banana Bites with Dark Chocolate

Smoothie: Peach and Ginger Smoothie with Flaxseed

**Day 28:**

Breakfast: Blueberry Almond Smoothie Bowl

Lunch: Caprese Salad with Basil Pesto

Dinner: Ratatouille with Herbed Quinoa

Snack: Zucchini Fritters with Greek Yogurt Sauce

Dessert: Lemon Blueberry Bars with Almond Crust

Smoothie: Raspberry and Almond Butter Smoothie

**Day 29:**

Breakfast: Apple Cinnamon Overnight Oats

Lunch: Roasted Vegetable and Quinoa Stuffed Bell Peppers

Dinner: Baked Cod with Tomato and Olive Relish

Snack: Stuffed Mushrooms with Spinach and Cheese

Dessert: Pumpkin Spice Energy Balls

Smoothie: Pineapple and Cucumber Smoothie with Mint

**Day 30:**

Breakfast: Veggie Packed Breakfast Burrito

Lunch: Greek-Style Chicken Wrap with Tzatziki Sauce

Dinner: Vegetarian Enchiladas with Black Beans and Sweet Potato

Snack: Mini Vegetable Quiches

Dessert: Mango and Coconut Rice Pudding

Smoothie: Coffee and Banana Smoothie with Oatmeal

# Chapter 2: Breakfast Recipes

Enjoy these delicious and nutritious breakfast recipes to kick-start your day on a healthy note!

## Hearty Oatmeal with Berries and Nuts

Ingredients:

- 1 cup rolled oats
- 2 cups water
- Pinch of salt
- 1/2 cup mixed berries (such as blueberries, raspberries, and strawberries)
- 2 tablespoons chopped nuts (such as almonds or walnuts)
- 1 tablespoon honey or maple syrup (optional)

Instructions:

1. In a saucepan, bring the water to a boil.

2. Add the rolled oats and salt to the boiling water, reduce the heat to low, and simmer for about 5 minutes, stirring occasionally.

3. Once the oatmeal reaches your desired consistency, remove it from the heat.

4. Transfer the oatmeal to serving bowls and top with mixed berries and chopped nuts.

5. Drizzle with honey or maple syrup, if desired.

6. Serve warm and enjoy a hearty and nutritious breakfast!

## Vegetable and Egg White Scramble

Ingredients:

- 4 egg whites
- 1/4 cup diced bell peppers (any color)
- 1/4 cup diced onion
- 1/4 cup diced tomatoes
- 1/4 cup chopped spinach
- Salt and pepper to taste
- 1 teaspoon olive oil

Instructions:

1. Heat the olive oil in a non-stick skillet over medium heat.

2. Add the diced bell peppers, onion, and tomatoes to the skillet and sauté for about 2-3 minutes until slightly softened.

3. Add the chopped spinach and cook for another minute until wilted.

4. In a bowl, whisk the egg whites with salt and pepper.

5. Pour the egg whites into the skillet with the vegetables.

6. Cook, stirring occasionally, until the egg whites are set and cooked through.

7. Remove from heat and transfer the scramble to a plate.

8. Serve hot and enjoy a delicious and protein-packed breakfast!

# Whole Wheat Pancakes with Sugar-Free Syrup

Ingredients:

- 1 cup whole wheat flour

- 1 tablespoon baking powder
- 1/4 teaspoon salt
- 1 tablespoon honey or maple syrup
- 1 cup almond milk (or any non-dairy milk)
- 1 teaspoon vanilla extract
- Cooking spray
- Sugar-free syrup for serving

Instructions:

1. In a mixing bowl, whisk together the whole wheat flour, baking powder, and salt.
2. In a separate bowl, mix the honey or maple syrup, almond milk, and vanilla extract.
3. Pour the wet ingredients into the dry ingredients and stir until just combined. Be careful not to overmix; a few lumps are fine.
4. Heat a non-stick skillet or griddle over medium heat and lightly coat with cooking spray.
5. Pour 1/4 cup of batter onto the skillet for each pancake.

6. Cook until bubbles form on the surface, then flip
   and cook for another 1-2 minutes until golden
   brown.

7. Repeat with the remaining batter.

8. Serve the pancakes with sugar-free syrup and enjoy
   a wholesome and satisfying breakfast!

## Greek Yogurt Parfait with Fresh Fruit

Ingredients:

- 1 cup plain Greek yogurt
- 1/4 cup granola
- 1/4 cup mixed fresh fruit (such as berries, sliced banana, or diced mango)
- 1 tablespoon honey (optional)

Instructions:

1. In a glass or bowl, layer half of the Greek yogurt.

2. Sprinkle half of the granola over the yogurt layer.

3. Add half of the mixed fresh fruit on top.

4. Repeat the layers with the remaining ingredients.

5. Drizzle with honey, if desired, for added sweetness.

6. Serve chilled and enjoy a refreshing and protein-rich breakfast parfait!

## Spinach and Mushroom Frittata

Ingredients:

- 4 large eggs
- 4 egg whites
- 1 cup baby spinach
- 1/2 cup sliced mushrooms
- 1/4 cup diced onion
- 1/4 cup shredded reduced-fat cheese (such as cheddar or mozzarella)
- Salt and pepper to taste
- Cooking spray

Instructions:

1. Preheat the oven to 350°F (175°C).
2. In a bowl, whisk together the eggs and egg whites. Season with salt and pepper.
3. Heat a non-stick skillet over medium heat and lightly coat with cooking spray.

4.  Add the diced onion and sliced mushrooms to the skillet and cook for 2-3 minutes until softened.

5.  Add the baby spinach to the skillet and cook for another minute until wilted.

6.  Pour the whisked eggs over the vegetables in the skillet.

7.  Sprinkle the shredded cheese evenly on top.

8.  Transfer the skillet to the preheated oven and bake for about 15-20 minutes until the frittata is set and golden brown on top.

9.  Remove from the oven and let it cool for a few minutes.

10. Slice into wedges and serve warm. Enjoy a flavorful and nutrient-packed frittata for breakfast!

## Quinoa Breakfast Bowl with Almonds and Cinnamon

Ingredients:

- 1/2 cup cooked quinoa
- 1/4 cup unsweetened almond milk (or any non-dairy milk)
- 1 tablespoon chopped almonds

- 1/2 teaspoon ground cinnamon

- 1 tablespoon honey or maple syrup (optional)

- Fresh berries for topping

Instructions:

1. In a bowl, combine the cooked quinoa, almond milk, chopped almonds, and ground cinnamon.

2. Stir well to combine all the ingredients.

3. Drizzle with honey or maple syrup, if desired, for added sweetness.

4. Top with fresh berries for a burst of flavor and color.

5. Serve at room temperature or chilled. Enjoy a nourishing and protein-rich quinoa breakfast bowl!

## Smoked Salmon and Avocado Toast

Ingredients:

- 2 slices whole wheat bread, toasted

- 2 ounces smoked salmon

- 1/2 avocado, sliced

- 1 tablespoon lemon juice

- 1 tablespoon chopped fresh dill

- Salt and pepper to taste

Instructions:

1. Mash the sliced avocado with lemon juice, chopped fresh dill, salt, and pepper in a small bowl.
2. Spread the mashed avocado mixture evenly on the toasted bread slices.
3. Top each slice with smoked salmon.
4. Garnish with additional dill, if desired.
5. Serve immediately and enjoy a delicious and satisfying smoked salmon and avocado toast for breakfast!

## Blueberry Almond Smoothie Bowl

Ingredients:

- 1 frozen banana
- 1/2 cup frozen blueberries
- 1/2 cup unsweetened almond milk (or any non-dairy milk)
- 1 tablespoon almond butter
- 1 tablespoon chia seeds

- Toppings: Fresh blueberries, sliced almonds, and granola

Instructions:

1. In a blender, combine the frozen banana, frozen blueberries, almond milk, almond butter, and chia seeds.
2. Blend until smooth and creamy.
3. Pour the smoothie into a bowl.
4. Top with fresh blueberries, sliced almonds, and granola for added texture and flavor.
5. Serve immediately and enjoy a refreshing and nutrient-packed blueberry almond smoothie bowl!

## Apple Cinnamon Overnight Oats

Ingredients:

- 1/2 cup rolled oats
- 1/2 cup unsweetened almond milk (or any non-dairy milk)
- 1/4 cup unsweetened applesauce
- 1/2 teaspoon ground cinnamon
- 1 tablespoon chopped walnuts

- 1 tablespoon maple syrup (optional)
- Sliced apple for garnish

Instructions:

1. In a jar or container, combine the rolled oats, almond milk, unsweetened applesauce, ground cinnamon, chopped walnuts, and maple syrup (if using).
2. Stir well to combine all the ingredients.
3. Cover the jar or container and refrigerate overnight or for at least 4-6 hours to allow the oats to absorb the liquid.
4. In the morning, give the oats a good stir.
5. Garnish with sliced apple for an extra crunch and flavor.
6. Enjoy the apple cinnamon overnight oats chilled for a convenient and nutritious breakfast!

## Veggie Packed Breakfast Burrito

Ingredients:

- 1 whole wheat tortilla
- 2 egg whites

- 1/4 cup diced bell peppers (any color)
- 1/4 cup diced onion
- 1/4 cup diced tomatoes
- 1/4 cup chopped spinach
- Salt and pepper to taste
- Salsa for serving

Instructions:

1. In a non-stick skillet, cook the diced bell peppers, onion, tomatoes, and chopped spinach over medium heat until softened.
2. Season with salt and pepper.
3. Add the egg whites to the skillet and cook, stirring occasionally, until set.
4. Warm the whole wheat tortilla in the microwave or on a stovetop.
5. Spoon the veggie and egg mixture onto the center of the tortilla.
6. Roll the tortilla tightly, tucking in the sides as you go.
7. Serve with salsa for added flavor and enjoy a wholesome and veggie-packed breakfast burrito!

# Chapter 3: Lunch Recipes

Enjoy these diverse and delicious lunch recipes. Each recipe is crafted with care to provide a balance of flavors and nutritious ingredients, making them ideal for maintaining a healthy lifestyle.

## Grilled Chicken and Vegetable Salad with Balsamic Vinaigrette

Ingredients:

- 2 boneless, skinless chicken breasts
- 1 tablespoon olive oil
- Salt and pepper to taste
- 4 cups mixed salad greens
- 1 cup cherry tomatoes, halved
- 1 cucumber, sliced
- 1 red onion, thinly sliced
- 1 avocado, sliced
- 1/4 cup crumbled feta cheese
- 2 tablespoons chopped fresh basil

Balsamic Vinaigrette:

- 3 tablespoons balsamic vinegar
- 1/4 cup extra virgin olive oil
- 1 teaspoon Dijon mustard
- 1 clove garlic, minced
- Salt and pepper to taste

Instructions:

1. Preheat the grill to medium-high heat.
2. Brush the chicken breasts with olive oil and season with salt and pepper.
3. Grill the chicken for 6-8 minutes per side, or until cooked through. Remove from the grill and let it rest for a few minutes. Slice the chicken into thin strips.
4. In a large salad bowl, combine the mixed greens, cherry tomatoes, cucumber, red onion, avocado, feta cheese, and chopped basil.
5. In a small bowl, whisk together the balsamic vinegar, olive oil, Dijon mustard, minced garlic, salt, and pepper to make the vinaigrette.

6. Drizzle the vinaigrette over the salad and toss to coat evenly.

7. Divide the salad onto plates and top with the grilled chicken slices.

8. Serve immediately and enjoy!

# Turkey and Hummus Wrap with Fresh Vegetables

Ingredients:

- 4 whole wheat tortillas
- 1/2 cup hummus
- 8 slices turkey breast
- 1 cup baby spinach leaves
- 1/2 cup shredded carrots
- 1/2 cup sliced cucumbers
- 1/4 cup sliced red bell pepper
- Salt and pepper to taste

Instructions:

1. Lay out the whole wheat tortillas on a clean surface.

2. Spread 2 tablespoons of hummus onto each tortilla, leaving a small border around the edges.

3. Place 2 slices of turkey breast on each tortilla, covering the hummus.

4. Top the turkey with a handful of baby spinach leaves, shredded carrots, sliced cucumbers, and sliced red bell pepper.

5. Season with salt and pepper to taste.

6. Roll up the tortillas tightly, tucking in the sides as you go.

7. Cut each wrap in half diagonally and secure with toothpicks, if desired.

8. Serve immediately or wrap tightly in foil or plastic wrap for later enjoyment.

## Quinoa and Black Bean Salad with Lime Dressing

Ingredients:

- 1 cup cooked quinoa
- 1 cup canned black beans, rinsed and drained
- 1 cup diced bell peppers (red, yellow, or orange)
- 1 cup corn kernels (fresh or frozen)
- 1/2 cup chopped fresh cilantro
- 1/4 cup diced red onion

- Juice of 2 limes
- 2 tablespoons extra virgin olive oil
- 1 clove garlic, minced
- Salt and pepper to taste

Instructions:

1. In a large bowl, combine the cooked quinoa, black beans, diced bell peppers, corn kernels, chopped cilantro, and diced red onion.
2. In a small bowl, whisk together the lime juice, olive oil, minced garlic, salt, and pepper to make the dressing.
3. Pour the dressing over the quinoa mixture and toss gently to combine.
4. Adjust the seasoning if needed.
5. Cover the bowl and refrigerate for at least 30 minutes to allow the flavors to meld.
6. Serve chilled as a refreshing salad or as a filling for wraps or tacos.

# Salmon and Quinoa Bowl with Lemon-Dill Dressing

Ingredients:

- 2 salmon fillets
- 2 tablespoons olive oil
- Salt and pepper to taste
- 2 cups cooked quinoa
- 2 cups mixed salad greens
- 1 cucumber, diced
- 1/2 cup cherry tomatoes, halved
- 1/4 cup chopped fresh dill
- Juice of 1 lemon
- 2 tablespoons Greek yogurt
- 1 clove garlic, minced

Instructions:

1. Preheat the oven to 400°F (200°C).
2. Place the salmon fillets on a baking sheet lined with parchment paper.
3. Drizzle the salmon with olive oil and season with salt and pepper.

4. Bake for 12-15 minutes, or until the salmon is cooked through and flakes easily with a fork.

5. Meanwhile, in a large bowl, combine the cooked quinoa, mixed salad greens, diced cucumber, and cherry tomatoes.

6. In a small bowl, whisk together the chopped dill, lemon juice, Greek yogurt, minced garlic, salt, and pepper to make the dressing.

7. Pour the dressing over the quinoa mixture and toss to coat evenly.

8. Divide the quinoa salad into bowls and top each with a baked salmon fillet.

9. Garnish with additional fresh dill if desired.

10. Serve immediately and enjoy the vibrant flavors.

## Mediterranean Chickpea Salad with Feta Cheese

Ingredients:

- 2 cups canned chickpeas, rinsed and drained
- 1 cup diced cucumber
- 1 cup halved cherry tomatoes
- 1/2 cup diced red onion

- 1/4 cup sliced Kalamata olives

- 1/4 cup crumbled feta cheese

- 2 tablespoons chopped fresh parsley

- 2 tablespoons extra virgin olive oil

- 1 tablespoon red wine vinegar

- 1 teaspoon dried oregano

- Salt and pepper to taste

Instructions:

1. In a large bowl, combine the chickpeas, diced cucumber, cherry tomatoes, diced red onion, Kalamata olives, crumbled feta cheese, and chopped parsley.

2. In a small bowl, whisk together the olive oil, red wine vinegar, dried oregano, salt, and pepper to make the dressing.

3. Pour the dressing over the chickpea mixture and toss gently to coat.

4. Adjust the seasoning if needed.

5. Cover the bowl and refrigerate for at least 30 minutes to allow the flavors to meld.

6.  Serve chilled as a refreshing salad or as a side dish
    to grilled meats or fish.

## Tofu Stir-Fry with Brown Rice

Ingredients:

- 1 block firm tofu, drained and cubed
- 2 tablespoons soy sauce
- 2 tablespoons hoisin sauce
- 1 tablespoon sesame oil
- 1 tablespoon cornstarch
- 1 tablespoon vegetable oil
- 2 cloves garlic, minced
- 1 teaspoon grated ginger
- 1 bell pepper, sliced
- 1 cup broccoli florets
- 1 carrot, sliced
- 1/2 cup snow peas
- 2 green onions, sliced
- Cooked brown rice for serving

Instructions:

1.  In a small bowl, whisk together the soy sauce, hoisin sauce, sesame oil, and cornstarch.

2.  Place the tofu cubes in a shallow dish and pour the sauce mixture over the tofu. Gently toss to coat the tofu evenly. Let it marinate for 10-15 minutes.

3.  Heat the vegetable oil in a large skillet or wok over medium-high heat.

4.  Add the minced garlic and grated ginger, and sauté for about 1 minute until fragrant.

5.  Add the marinated tofu to the skillet and cook for 4-5 minutes, stirring occasionally, until the tofu is lightly browned.

6.  Add the sliced bell pepper, broccoli florets, carrot slices, and snow peas to the skillet. Stir-fry for an additional 5-6 minutes, or until the vegetables are tender-crisp.

7.  Stir in the sliced green onions and cook for another minute.

8.  Serve the tofu stir-fry over cooked brown rice and enjoy a flavorful and nutritious lunch.

# Lentil Soup with Spinach and Tomatoes

Ingredients:

- 1 cup dried green lentils
- 1 tablespoon olive oil
- 1 onion, diced
- 2 cloves garlic, minced
- 2 carrots, diced
- 2 celery stalks, diced
- 1 can diced tomatoes (14 oz/400 g)
- 4 cups vegetable broth
- 2 cups fresh spinach leaves
- 1 teaspoon dried thyme
- 1/2 teaspoon dried oregano
- Salt and pepper to taste

Instructions:

1. Rinse the dried lentils under cold water and drain.
2. In a large pot, heat the olive oil over medium heat.
3. Add the diced onion and minced garlic, and sauté for 2-3 minutes until fragrant.

4. Add the diced carrots and celery, and cook for another 5 minutes, stirring occasionally.

5. Stir in the canned diced tomatoes (including the juice) and the drained lentils.

6. Pour in the vegetable broth and add the dried thyme and oregano.

7. Bring the soup to a boil, then reduce the heat and simmer for about 30-40 minutes, or until the lentils are tender.

8. Stir in the fresh spinach leaves and cook for an additional 5 minutes, or until wilted.

9. Season with salt and pepper to taste.

10. Ladle the lentil soup into bowls and serve hot. Enjoy this comforting and nutritious lunch option.

## Caprese Salad with Basil Pesto

Ingredients:

- 2 large ripe tomatoes, sliced
- 1/2 pound fresh mozzarella cheese, sliced
- 1/4 cup fresh basil leaves
- 2 tablespoons extra virgin olive oil
- 2 tablespoons balsamic vinegar

- Salt and pepper to taste
- Basil pesto for drizzling (store-bought or homemade)

Instructions:

1. Arrange the tomato slices and mozzarella slices on a serving platter, alternating them.
2. Place the fresh basil leaves on top of each tomato and mozzarella slice.
3. Drizzle the extra virgin olive oil and balsamic vinegar over the salad.
4. Season with salt and pepper to taste.
5. Just before serving, drizzle the basil pesto over the Caprese salad.
6. Serve as a light and refreshing lunch or as a side dish to complement your main course.

## Roasted Vegetable and Quinoa Stuffed Bell Peppers

Ingredients:

- 4 bell peppers (any color)
- 1 cup cooked quinoa

- 1 zucchini, diced

- 1 yellow squash, diced

- 1 red onion, diced

- 1 cup cherry tomatoes, halved

- 2 cloves garlic, minced

- 2 tablespoons extra virgin olive oil

- 1 teaspoon dried basil

- 1/2 teaspoon dried oregano

- Salt and pepper to taste

- Grated Parmesan cheese for topping (optional)

Instructions:

1. Preheat the oven to 400°F (200°C).

2. Slice off the tops of the bell peppers and remove the seeds and membranes.

3. In a large bowl, combine the cooked quinoa, diced zucchini, diced yellow squash, diced red onion, cherry tomatoes, minced garlic, extra virgin olive oil, dried basil, dried oregano, salt, and pepper. Toss to coat the vegetables and quinoa evenly.

4. Stuff the bell peppers with the quinoa and vegetable mixture, packing them tightly.

5. Place the stuffed bell peppers in a baking dish and cover with foil.

6. Bake for 25-30 minutes, or until the peppers are tender and the filling is heated through.

7. Remove the foil and sprinkle grated Parmesan cheese on top of each stuffed pepper if desired.

8. Return to the oven for an additional 5 minutes to melt the cheese.

9. Serve the roasted vegetable and quinoa stuffed bell peppers as a delicious and wholesome lunch option.

## Greek-Style Chicken Wrap with Tzatziki Sauce

Ingredients:

- 2 boneless, skinless chicken breasts
- 2 tablespoons Greek seasoning blend
- 1 tablespoon olive oil
- Salt and pepper to taste
- 4 whole wheat tortillas
- 1/2 cup tzatziki sauce
- 1 cup chopped romaine lettuce
- 1/2 cup sliced cucumber

- 1/4 cup sliced red onion
- 1/4 cup crumbled feta cheese

Instructions:

1. Preheat the grill or grill pan to medium-high heat.
2. Season the chicken breasts with Greek seasoning, olive oil, salt, and pepper, ensuring they are evenly coated.
3. Grill the chicken for about 6-8 minutes per side, or until cooked through. Let it rest for a few minutes, then slice it into thin strips.
4. Lay out the whole wheat tortillas on a clean surface.
5. Spread 2 tablespoons of tzatziki sauce onto each tortilla, leaving a small border around the edges.
6. Divide the sliced grilled chicken, chopped romaine lettuce, sliced cucumber, sliced red onion, and crumbled feta cheese among the tortillas.
7. Roll up the tortillas tightly, tucking in the sides as you go.
8. Cut each wrap in half diagonally and secure with toothpicks, if desired.

9.  Serve the Greek-style chicken wraps as a flavorful
    and satisfying lunch option.

# Chapter 4: Dinner Recipes

As we dive into a delectable collection of nutritious and scrumptious dinner recipes that are not only heart-healthy but also diabetes-friendly. These dishes are designed to tantalize your taste buds while promoting a balanced and wholesome diet to support your health and well-being.

## Grilled Salmon with Lemon and Dill

Ingredients:

- 4 salmon fillets
- 2 tablespoons olive oil
- 2 tablespoons freshly squeezed lemon juice
- 1 tablespoon fresh dill, chopped
- 2 cloves garlic, minced
- Salt and pepper to taste
- Lemon slices for garnish

Instructions:

1. Preheat your grill to medium-high heat.

2. In a small bowl, whisk together the olive oil, lemon juice, minced garlic, chopped dill, salt, and pepper.

3. Place the salmon fillets in a shallow dish and pour the marinade over them. Ensure each fillet is evenly coated with the marinade. Let it marinate for about 20-30 minutes.

4. Grease the grill grates lightly with oil to prevent sticking.

5. Place the marinated salmon fillets on the grill and cook for about 4-5 minutes on each side or until the fish flakes easily with a fork.

6. Once cooked, remove the salmon from the grill and garnish with lemon slices.

7. Serve the grilled salmon with a side of steamed vegetables or a refreshing mixed green salad.

## Baked Chicken Breast with Herbs and Garlic

Ingredients:

- 4 boneless, skinless chicken breasts
- 2 tablespoons olive oil
- 2 cloves garlic, minced

- 1 teaspoon dried thyme
- 1 teaspoon dried rosemary
- 1 teaspoon dried oregano
- Salt and pepper to taste

Instructions:

1. Preheat your oven to 375°F (190°C).
2. In a small bowl, mix together the olive oil, minced garlic, dried thyme, dried rosemary, dried oregano, salt, and pepper.
3. Place the chicken breasts in a baking dish and brush the herb and garlic mixture over each piece, making sure to coat them thoroughly.
4. Bake the chicken in the preheated oven for approximately 25-30 minutes or until the internal temperature reaches 165°F (74°C) and the chicken is cooked through.
5. Once done, remove the baked chicken from the oven and let it rest for a few minutes before serving.
6. Pair the flavorful baked chicken with a side of steamed vegetables or quinoa for a complete and satisfying meal.

# Shrimp and Broccoli Stir-Fry with Brown Rice

Ingredients:

- 1 lb (450g) shrimp, peeled and deveined
- 2 cups broccoli florets
- 1 red bell pepper, thinly sliced
- 1 carrot, julienned
- 3 tablespoons low-sodium soy sauce
- 2 tablespoons hoisin sauce
- 1 tablespoon sesame oil
- 2 cloves garlic, minced
- 1 teaspoon fresh ginger, grated
- 2 tablespoons olive oil
- 3 cups cooked brown rice

Instructions:

1. In a small bowl, combine the low-sodium soy sauce, hoisin sauce, sesame oil, minced garlic, and grated ginger. Set aside.
2. Heat the olive oil in a large skillet or wok over medium-high heat.

3. Add the shrimp to the skillet and stir-fry for 2-3 minutes until they turn pink and opaque. Remove the shrimp from the skillet and set aside.

4. In the same skillet, add the broccoli florets, red bell pepper slices, and julienned carrot. Stir-fry for about 4-5 minutes until the vegetables are crisp-tender.

5. Return the cooked shrimp to the skillet and pour the sauce mixture over the shrimp and vegetables. Stir to coat everything evenly and cook for an additional 1-2 minutes until heated through.

6. Serve the shrimp and broccoli stir-fry over a bed of cooked brown rice for a wholesome and satisfying meal.

## Turkey Chili with Beans and Veggies

Ingredients:

- 1 lb (450g) lean ground turkey
- 1 onion, diced
- 2 cloves garlic, minced
- 1 bell pepper, diced
- 1 zucchini, diced

- 1 can (14 oz) diced tomatoes

- 1 can (14 oz) kidney beans, rinsed and drained

- 1 can (14 oz) black beans, rinsed and drained

- 1 cup low-sodium chicken broth

- 2 tablespoons chili powder

- 1 teaspoon cumin

- 1 teaspoon paprika

- Salt and pepper to taste

- Optional toppings: shredded cheese, chopped green onions, Greek yogurt

Instructions:

1. In a large pot or Dutch oven, cook the ground turkey over medium heat until browned. Drain any excess fat if necessary.

2. Add the diced onion, minced garlic, diced bell pepper, and diced zucchini to the pot. Cook for about 5 minutes until the vegetables have softened.

3. Stir in the diced tomatoes, kidney beans, black beans, chicken broth, chili powder, cumin, paprika, salt, and pepper. Bring the mixture to a boil.

4. Reduce the heat to low, cover the pot, and let the chili simmer for about 30-40 minutes to allow the flavors to meld together.

5. Taste the chili and adjust the seasonings as desired.

6. Serve the turkey chili hot and garnish with shredded cheese, chopped green onions, or a dollop of Greek yogurt, if desired. This hearty and flavorful chili pairs well with whole grain bread or brown rice.

## Spinach and Feta Stuffed Chicken Breast

Ingredients:

- 4 boneless, skinless chicken breasts
- 2 cups fresh spinach leaves
- 1/2 cup crumbled feta cheese
- 2 cloves garlic, minced
- 1 tablespoon olive oil
- Salt and pepper to taste

Instructions:

1. Preheat your oven to 400°F (200°C).

2. Using a sharp knife, cut a pocket horizontally into each chicken breast, being careful not to cut through the other side.

3. In a skillet, heat the olive oil over medium heat. Add the minced garlic and cook for about 1 minute until fragrant.

4. Add the fresh spinach leaves to the skillet and sauté until wilted, approximately 2-3 minutes.

5. Remove the skillet from heat and stir in the crumbled feta cheese. Season with salt and pepper to taste.

6. Stuff each chicken breast with the spinach and feta mixture, dividing it equally among the breasts. Secure the openings with toothpicks if needed.

7. Place the stuffed chicken breasts in a baking dish and bake in the preheated oven for 25-30 minutes or until the chicken is cooked through and no longer pink in the center.

8. Remove the toothpicks before serving. Pair the spinach and feta stuffed chicken breast with a side of roasted vegetables or a quinoa salad for a wholesome and satisfying dinner.

# Eggplant and Chickpea Curry with Brown Rice

Ingredients:

- 1 large eggplant, diced
- 1 can (14 oz) chickpeas, rinsed and drained
- 1 onion, diced
- 3 cloves garlic, minced
- 1 can (14 oz) diced tomatoes
- 1 can (14 oz) coconut milk
- 2 tablespoons curry powder
- 1 teaspoon cumin
- 1 teaspoon turmeric
- 1/2 teaspoon cinnamon
- Salt and pepper to taste
- Fresh cilantro for garnish
- Cooked brown rice for serving

Instructions:

1. Heat a tablespoon of olive oil in a large pot or skillet over medium heat.
2. Add the diced eggplant and cook for 5-6 minutes until it starts to soften.

3. Add the diced onion and minced garlic to the pot and cook for an additional 2-3 minutes until the onion becomes translucent.

4. Stir in the curry powder, cumin, turmeric, cinnamon, salt, and pepper. Cook for 1 minute until fragrant.

5. Add the chickpeas, diced tomatoes, and coconut milk to the pot. Stir well to combine all the ingredients.

6. Reduce the heat to low, cover the pot, and let the curry simmer for 20-25 minutes, allowing the flavors to meld together and the eggplant to become tender.

7. Taste the curry and adjust the seasonings if needed.

8. Serve the eggplant and chickpea curry hot over cooked brown rice. Garnish with fresh cilantro for added freshness and flavor.

## Beef and Vegetable Stir-Fry with Quinoa

Ingredients:

- 1 lb (450g) beef sirloin, thinly sliced

- 2 tablespoons low-sodium soy sauce

- 2 tablespoons hoisin sauce

- 1 tablespoon cornstarch

- 1 tablespoon olive oil

- 2 cloves garlic, minced

- 1 bell pepper, thinly sliced

- 1 cup broccoli florets

- 1 carrot, julienned

- 1 cup snow peas

- 2 green onions, sliced

- 2 cups cooked quinoa

Instructions:

1. In a small bowl, whisk together the low-sodium soy sauce, hoisin sauce, and cornstarch until smooth. Set aside.

2. Heat the olive oil in a large skillet or wok over high heat.

3. Add the minced garlic and sliced beef to the skillet. Stir-fry for 2-3 minutes until the beef is browned and cooked to your desired doneness. Remove the beef from the skillet and set aside.

4.  In the same skillet, add the bell pepper slices, broccoli florets, julienned carrot, and snow peas. Stir-fry for about 4-5 minutes until the vegetables are crisp-tender.

5.  Return the cooked beef to the skillet and pour the sauce mixture over the beef and vegetables. Stir well to coat everything evenly and cook for an additional 1-2 minutes until the sauce thickens.

6.  Remove the skillet from heat and garnish the stir-fry with sliced green onions.

7.  Serve the beef and vegetable stir-fry over a bed of cooked quinoa for a nutritious and satisfying meal.

## Ratatouille with Herbed Quinoa

Ingredients:

- 1 eggplant, diced
- 1 zucchini, diced
- 1 yellow squash, diced
- 1 red bell pepper, diced
- 1 onion, diced
- 3 cloves garlic, minced
- 2 tablespoons olive oil

- 1 can (14 oz) diced tomatoes
- 1 tablespoon tomato paste
- 1 teaspoon dried thyme
- 1 teaspoon dried rosemary
- Salt and pepper to taste
- Fresh basil for garnish
- Herbed quinoa (recipe follows)

Instructions:

1. In a large pot or Dutch oven, heat the olive oil over medium heat.
2. Add the diced onion and minced garlic to the pot. Cook for 2-3 minutes until the onion becomes translucent.
3. Stir in the diced eggplant, zucchini, yellow squash, and red bell pepper. Cook for about 5 minutes until the vegetables start to soften.
4. Add the diced tomatoes, tomato paste, dried thyme, dried rosemary, salt, and pepper to the pot. Stir well to combine all the ingredients.
5. Reduce the heat to low, cover the pot, and let the ratatouille simmer for 30-40 minutes, allowing the

flavors to meld together and the vegetables to
become tender.

6.  Taste the ratatouille and adjust the seasonings if
    needed.

7.  Serve the ratatouille hot, garnished with fresh basil,
    alongside a portion of herbed quinoa.

Herbed Quinoa:

Ingredients:

- 1 cup quinoa
- 2 cups low-sodium vegetable broth
- 1 tablespoon chopped fresh parsley
- 1 tablespoon chopped fresh basil
- 1 tablespoon chopped fresh thyme
- Salt and pepper to taste

Instructions:

1.  Rinse the quinoa under cold water to remove any
    bitter coating.

2.  In a saucepan, combine the rinsed quinoa and
    vegetable broth. Bring to a boil over medium-high
    heat.

3. Reduce the heat to low, cover the saucepan, and let the quinoa simmer for 15-20 minutes until the liquid is absorbed and the quinoa is tender.

4. Remove the saucepan from heat and let the quinoa sit covered for 5 minutes.

5. Fluff the quinoa with a fork and stir in the chopped fresh parsley, basil, thyme, salt, and pepper.

## Baked Cod with Tomato and Olive Relish

Ingredients:

- 4 cod fillets
- 2 tablespoons olive oil
- 2 cloves garlic, minced
- 1 teaspoon dried oregano
- 1/2 teaspoon paprika
- Salt and pepper to taste
- Tomato and Olive Relish:
- 1 cup cherry tomatoes, halved
- 1/4 cup sliced Kalamata olives
- 1 tablespoon chopped fresh basil
- 1 tablespoon chopped fresh parsley

- 1 tablespoon balsamic vinegar

- 1 tablespoon olive oil

- Salt and pepper to taste

Instructions:

1. Preheat your oven to 400°F (200°C).

2. Place the cod fillets in a baking dish.

3. In a small bowl, whisk together the olive oil, minced garlic, dried oregano, paprika, salt, and pepper.

4. Brush the olive oil mixture over the cod fillets, ensuring they are evenly coated.

5. Bake the cod in the preheated oven for approximately 12-15 minutes until the fish is opaque and flakes easily with a fork.

6. While the cod is baking, prepare the tomato and olive relish. In a bowl, combine the halved cherry tomatoes, sliced Kalamata olives, chopped fresh basil, chopped fresh parsley, balsamic vinegar, olive oil, salt, and pepper. Toss gently to mix.

7. Once the cod is cooked, remove it from the oven and top each fillet with a generous spoonful of the tomato and olive relish.

8. Serve the baked cod with the flavorful tomato and olive relish alongside a side of steamed vegetables or a quinoa salad for a satisfying dinner.

## Vegetarian Enchiladas with Black Beans and Sweet Potato

Ingredients:

- 1 tablespoon olive oil

- 1 onion, diced

- 2 cloves garlic, minced

- 1 sweet potato, peeled and diced

- 1 can (14 oz) black beans, rinsed and drained

- 1 can (4 oz) diced green chilies

- 1 can (14 oz) enchilada sauce

- 1 teaspoon ground cumin

- 1/2 teaspoon chili powder

- Salt and pepper to taste

- 8 small flour tortillas

- 1 cup shredded Mexican cheese blend

- Optional toppings: chopped fresh cilantro, diced avocado, sour cream

Instructions:

1. Preheat your oven to 375°F (190°C).
2. In a large skillet, heat the olive oil over medium heat.
3. Add the diced onion and minced garlic to the skillet. Cook for 2-3 minutes until the onion becomes translucent.
4. Stir in the diced sweet potato, black beans, diced green chilies, ground cumin, chili powder, salt, and pepper. Cook for about 5 minutes until the sweet potato starts to soften.
5. Pour half of the enchilada sauce into the skillet and stir well to coat the sweet potato and bean mixture.
6. Spoon a generous portion of the filling onto each flour tortilla, roll it up tightly, and place it seam-side down in a greased baking dish.
7. Pour the remaining enchilada sauce over the rolled tortillas, ensuring they are fully covered.

8.  Sprinkle the shredded Mexican cheese blend evenly over the enchiladas.

9.  Cover the baking dish with foil and bake in the preheated oven for 20-25 minutes until the enchiladas are heated through and the cheese is melted and bubbly.

10. Remove the foil and bake for an additional 5 minutes to allow the cheese to slightly brown.

11. Serve the vegetarian enchiladas hot with your choice of optional toppings, such as chopped fresh cilantro, diced avocado, or sour cream. These flavorful and satisfying enchiladas pair well with a side of Mexican rice or a refreshing green salad.

# Chapter 5: Snacks and Appetizers

Enjoy these delicious and healthy snacks and appetizers

## Roasted Red Pepper Hummus with Veggie Sticks

Ingredients:

- 1 can (15 ounces) chickpeas, drained and rinsed
- 2 roasted red peppers, peeled and seeded
- 3 tablespoons tahini
- 2 cloves garlic, minced
- 2 tablespoons lemon juice
- 2 tablespoons olive oil
- 1/2 teaspoon cumin
- Salt and pepper to taste
- Assorted vegetable sticks (carrots, celery, bell peppers) for serving

Instructions:

1. In a food processor, combine the chickpeas, roasted red peppers, tahini, minced garlic, lemon juice, olive oil, cumin, salt, and pepper.

2. Blend until smooth and creamy, scraping down the sides as needed.

3. Taste and adjust the seasonings if necessary.

4. Transfer the hummus to a serving bowl and garnish with a drizzle of olive oil and a sprinkle of cumin, if desired.

5. Serve with assorted vegetable sticks for dipping.

## Baked Sweet Potato Chips with Yogurt Dip

Ingredients:

- 2 large sweet potatoes, peeled
- 2 tablespoons olive oil
- 1 teaspoon paprika
- 1/2 teaspoon garlic powder
- Salt and pepper to taste
- 1 cup Greek yogurt
- 1 tablespoon lemon juice
- 1 tablespoon chopped fresh dill

- 1 clove garlic, minced

Instructions:

1. Preheat the oven to 375°F (190°C) and line two baking sheets with parchment paper.
2. Slice the sweet potatoes into thin rounds using a mandoline slicer or a sharp knife.
3. In a large bowl, toss the sweet potato slices with olive oil, paprika, garlic powder, salt, and pepper until evenly coated.
4. Arrange the sweet potato slices in a single layer on the prepared baking sheets.
5. Bake for 15-20 minutes, flipping the chips halfway through, until they are crispy and golden brown.
6. Meanwhile, in a small bowl, whisk together the Greek yogurt, lemon juice, chopped dill, and minced garlic to make the dip.
7. Season the dip with salt and pepper to taste.
8. Once the sweet potato chips are done, remove them from the oven and let them cool for a few minutes.
9. Serve the baked sweet potato chips with the yogurt dip on the side.

# Avocado and Tomato Salsa with Whole Wheat Pita Chips

Ingredients:

- 2 ripe avocados, diced
- 1 cup cherry tomatoes, halved
- 1/4 cup red onion, finely chopped
- 1 jalapeño pepper, seeded and minced
- 2 tablespoons fresh cilantro, chopped
- 2 tablespoons lime juice
- Salt and pepper to taste
- Whole wheat pita bread, cut into triangles, for serving

Instructions:

1. In a medium bowl, combine the diced avocados, cherry tomatoes, red onion, jalapeño pepper, cilantro, and lime juice.
2. Gently toss the ingredients together until well mixed.
3. Season with salt and pepper to taste.
4. Cover the bowl with plastic wrap and refrigerate for at least 30 minutes to allow the flavors to meld.

5. Preheat the oven to 350°F (175°C).

6. Arrange the whole wheat pita triangles on a baking sheet in a single layer.

7. Bake for 8-10 minutes, or until the pita chips are crisp and lightly golden.

8. Remove the pita chips from the oven and let them cool.

9. Serve the avocado and tomato salsa with the whole wheat pita chips for dipping.

## Greek Yogurt and Berry Popsicles

Ingredients:

- 1 cup Greek yogurt
- 1 cup mixed berries (strawberries, blueberries, raspberries)
- 2 tablespoons honey (optional)

Instructions:

1. In a blender or food processor, combine the Greek yogurt, mixed berries, and honey (if using).

2. Blend until smooth and well combined.

3. Taste the mixture and add more honey if desired for added sweetness.

4. Pour the mixture into popsicle molds, leaving a little space at the top for expansion.

5. Insert popsicle sticks into the molds and freeze for at least 4 hours, or until the popsicles are completely frozen.

6. To remove the popsicles from the molds, run warm water over the bottom of the molds for a few seconds to loosen them.

7. Gently pull the popsicles out and serve immediately.

## Cucumber and Tuna Bites

Ingredients:

- 1 English cucumber
- 1 can (5 ounces) tuna, drained
- 2 tablespoons mayonnaise
- 1 tablespoon chopped fresh dill
- 1 tablespoon lemon juice
- Salt and pepper to taste

Instructions:

1.  Cut the cucumber into thick rounds, about 1/2 inch thick.

2.  Use a small spoon or melon baller to scoop out the center of each cucumber round, creating a small well.

3.  In a bowl, mix together the drained tuna, mayonnaise, chopped dill, lemon juice, salt, and pepper.

4.  Spoon a small amount of the tuna mixture into each cucumber well, pressing it down slightly.

5.  Arrange the cucumber and tuna bites on a serving platter.

6.  Garnish with additional dill, if desired.

7.  Serve chilled.

## Spiced Nuts and Seeds Mix

Ingredients:

- 1 cup mixed nuts (almonds, cashews, walnuts)
- 1/4 cup pumpkin seeds
- 1/4 cup sunflower seeds
- 1 tablespoon olive oil

- 1 tablespoon honey
- 1/2 teaspoon ground cumin
- 1/2 teaspoon ground paprika
- 1/4 teaspoon cayenne pepper (optional)
- Salt to taste

Instructions:

1. Preheat the oven to 325°F (160°C) and line a baking sheet with parchment paper.
2. In a bowl, combine the mixed nuts, pumpkin seeds, sunflower seeds, olive oil, honey, cumin, paprika, cayenne pepper (if using), and salt.
3. Toss the mixture until the nuts and seeds are evenly coated with the spices and honey.
4. Spread the mixture in a single layer on the prepared baking sheet.
5. Bake for 15-20 minutes, stirring once or twice, until the nuts and seeds are golden brown and fragrant.
6. Remove from the oven and let the spiced nuts and seeds mix cool completely.
7. Once cooled, transfer to an airtight container for storage.

8. Serve as a healthy and flavorful snack.

## Edamame and Sea Salt

Ingredients:

- 2 cups frozen edamame, thawed
- Sea salt to taste

Instructions:

1. Bring a pot of water to a boil.
2. Add the thawed edamame to the boiling water and cook for 3-5 minutes, or until tender.
3. Drain the edamame and rinse with cold water to stop the cooking process.
4. Sprinkle with sea salt to taste.
5. Serve the edamame as a nutritious and satisfying snack.

## Zucchini Fritters with Greek Yogurt Sauce

Ingredients:

- 2 medium zucchini, grated

- 1/2 teaspoon salt

- 1/4 cup grated Parmesan cheese

- 1/4 cup breadcrumbs

- 1 clove garlic, minced

- 1 egg, beaten

- 2 tablespoons chopped fresh parsley

- 1 tablespoon chopped fresh dill

- 1/4 teaspoon black pepper

- Olive oil for frying

Greek Yogurt Sauce:

- 1/2 cup Greek yogurt

- 1 tablespoon lemon juice

- 1 tablespoon chopped fresh dill

- Salt and pepper to taste

Instructions:

1. Place the grated zucchini in a colander and sprinkle with salt.

2. Let it sit for 10-15 minutes to release excess moisture.

3.  Squeeze the zucchini to remove as much liquid as possible and transfer it to a clean kitchen towel.

4.  Wrap the zucchini in the towel and squeeze again to remove any remaining moisture.

5.  In a large bowl, combine the grated zucchini, Parmesan cheese, breadcrumbs, minced garlic, beaten egg, chopped parsley, chopped dill, and black pepper.

6.  Mix until well combined.

7.  Heat a thin layer of olive oil in a skillet over medium heat.

8.  Spoon the zucchini mixture into the skillet, forming small fritters about 2-3 inches in diameter.

9.  Cook the fritters for 3-4 minutes per side, or until golden brown and crispy.

10. Remove the fritters from the skillet and place them on a paper towel-lined plate to absorb any excess oil.

11. In a small bowl, mix together the Greek yogurt, lemon juice, chopped dill, salt, and pepper to make the sauce.

12. Serve the zucchini fritters with the Greek yogurt sauce on the side.

## Stuffed Mushrooms with Spinach and Cheese

Ingredients:

- 12 large button mushrooms
- 1 tablespoon olive oil
- 1/2 onion, finely chopped
- 2 cloves garlic, minced
- 2 cups fresh spinach, chopped
- 1/4 cup grated Parmesan cheese
- 1/4 cup breadcrumbs
- Salt and pepper to taste

Instructions:

1. Preheat the oven to 375°F (190°C) and line a baking sheet with parchment paper.
2. Remove the stems from the mushrooms and set them aside.
3. Arrange the mushroom caps on the prepared baking sheet.
4. In a skillet, heat the olive oil over medium heat.

5.  Add the chopped onion and minced garlic to the skillet and sauté until the onion is translucent.

6.  Add the chopped mushroom stems and cook for an additional 2-3 minutes.

7.  Stir in the chopped spinach and cook until wilted.

8.  Remove the skillet from the heat and let the mixture cool slightly.

9.  Stir in the grated Parmesan cheese, breadcrumbs, salt, and pepper.

10. Spoon the spinach and cheese mixture into each mushroom cap, filling them generously.

11. Bake the stuffed mushrooms in the preheated oven for 15-20 minutes, or until the mushrooms are tender and the filling is golden brown.

12. Remove from the oven and let the stuffed mushrooms cool for a few minutes before serving.

## Mini Vegetable Quiches

Ingredients:

- 1 cup mixed vegetables (bell peppers, broccoli, mushrooms), chopped
- 1/2 onion, finely chopped

- 1 clove garlic, minced
- 1 tablespoon olive oil
- 4 large eggs
- 1/2 cup milk
- 1/4 cup grated cheddar cheese
- Salt and pepper to taste

Instructions:

1. Preheat the oven to 375°F (190°C) and grease a muffin tin.
2. In a skillet, heat the olive oil over medium heat.
3. Add the chopped onion and minced garlic to the skillet and sauté until the onion is translucent.
4. Add the mixed vegetables to the skillet and cook until they are tender.
5. In a bowl, whisk together the eggs, milk, grated cheddar cheese, salt, and pepper.
6. Divide the sautéed vegetables evenly among the greased muffin cups.
7. Pour the egg mixture over the vegetables, filling each cup about three-quarters full.

8.  Bake in the preheated oven for 20-25 minutes, or until the quiches are set and golden brown on top.

9.  Remove from the oven and let the mini vegetable quiches cool for a few minutes before removing them from the muffin tin.

10. Serve warm or at room temperature.

# Chapter 6: Desserts

## Fresh Berry Parfait with Whipped Cream

Ingredients:

- 1 cup mixed fresh berries (strawberries, blueberries, raspberries)
- 1 cup low-fat Greek yogurt
- 2 tablespoons honey
- 1 teaspoon vanilla extract
- 1 cup whipped cream
- Fresh mint leaves for garnish

Instructions:

1. Rinse the fresh berries under cold water and pat them dry with a paper towel.
2. In a medium bowl, combine the Greek yogurt, honey, and vanilla extract. Stir well to incorporate.
3. Take serving glasses or parfait dishes and start layering the ingredients. Begin with a spoonful of

the Greek yogurt mixture at the bottom of each glass.

4. Add a layer of mixed berries on top of the yogurt.

5. Continue alternating between layers of yogurt and berries until the glasses are filled, finishing with a layer of berries on top.

6. Top each parfait with a dollop of whipped cream.

7. Garnish with fresh mint leaves.

8. Refrigerate for at least 30 minutes to allow the flavors to meld together.

9. Serve chilled and enjoy!

## Chocolate Avocado Mousse

Ingredients:

- 2 ripe avocados
- 1/4 cup unsweetened cocoa powder
- 1/4 cup honey or maple syrup
- 1 teaspoon vanilla extract
- Pinch of salt
- Fresh berries for garnish

Instructions:

1. Cut the avocados in half, remove the pit, and scoop out the flesh into a blender or food processor.

2. Add the cocoa powder, honey or maple syrup, vanilla extract, and a pinch of salt to the blender.

3. Blend the ingredients until smooth and creamy, scraping down the sides as needed.

4. Taste the mousse and adjust the sweetness if desired by adding more honey or maple syrup.

5. Transfer the mousse to serving bowls or glasses.

6. Cover and refrigerate for at least 1 hour to chill and set.

7. Before serving, garnish each portion with fresh berries.

8. Serve chilled and indulge in this rich and decadent chocolate avocado mousse!

## Greek Yogurt and Fruit Popsicles

Ingredients:

- 1 cup plain Greek yogurt
- 2 tablespoons honey or agave syrup
- 1 teaspoon vanilla extract

- 1 cup mixed fresh fruit (strawberries, blueberries, diced peaches, etc.)
- Popsicle molds
- Popsicle sticks

Instructions:

1. In a bowl, combine the Greek yogurt, honey or agave syrup, and vanilla extract. Mix well until smooth.
2. Prepare the fresh fruit by washing, cutting, and dicing into small pieces.
3. Fill each popsicle mold halfway with the Greek yogurt mixture.
4. Add a spoonful of mixed fresh fruit to each mold, pressing it down gently.
5. Continue layering the yogurt and fruit until the molds are full, leaving a small space at the top to allow for expansion.
6. Insert a popsicle stick into each mold, making sure it is centered.
7. Place the molds in the freezer and freeze for at least 4 hours or until solid.

8. To remove the popsicles from the molds, run them briefly under warm water to loosen.

9. Enjoy these refreshing and nutritious Greek yogurt and fruit popsicles on a hot day!

## Baked Apple with Cinnamon and Walnuts

Ingredients:

- 2 apples (preferably Granny Smith or Honeycrisp)
- 2 tablespoons chopped walnuts
- 1 tablespoon honey or maple syrup
- 1 teaspoon ground cinnamon
- 1/4 teaspoon nutmeg
- 1 tablespoon unsalted butter, melted
- Vanilla ice cream or Greek yogurt for serving (optional)

Instructions:

1. Preheat the oven to 375°F (190°C).
2. Core the apples using an apple corer or a small knife, leaving the bottoms intact.

3. In a small bowl, combine the chopped walnuts, honey or maple syrup, ground cinnamon, and nutmeg. Mix well.

4. Stuff each apple with the walnut mixture, packing it tightly into the cavity.

5. Place the stuffed apples in a baking dish and drizzle the melted butter over them.

6. Bake in the preheated oven for 25-30 minutes or until the apples are tender and the filling is golden brown.

7. Remove from the oven and let the apples cool slightly.

8. Serve the baked apples as is or with a scoop of vanilla ice cream or a dollop of Greek yogurt, if desired.

9. Enjoy the warm, fragrant flavors of this comforting baked apple dessert!

# Mixed Berry Crumble with Oat Topping

Ingredients:

- 2 cups mixed berries (strawberries, blueberries, raspberries)
- 1/4 cup granulated sugar
- 1 tablespoon lemon juice
- 1/2 cup all-purpose flour
- 1/2 cup rolled oats
- 1/4 cup brown sugar
- 1/4 teaspoon ground cinnamon
- Pinch of salt
- 4 tablespoons unsalted butter, chilled and cubed

Instructions:

1. Preheat the oven to 375°F (190°C).
2. In a bowl, combine the mixed berries, granulated sugar, and lemon juice. Toss gently to coat the berries with the sugar and lemon juice.
3. Transfer the berry mixture to a baking dish or individual ramekins, spreading it out evenly.

4.  In a separate bowl, combine the flour, rolled oats, brown sugar, ground cinnamon, and salt.

5.  Add the chilled cubed butter to the dry ingredients and use your fingers or a pastry cutter to mix until the mixture resembles coarse crumbs.

6.  Sprinkle the oat topping evenly over the berry mixture in the baking dish.

7.  Place the dish in the preheated oven and bake for 25-30 minutes or until the topping is golden brown and the berries are bubbling.

8.  Remove from the oven and let the crumble cool for a few minutes before serving.

9.  Serve the mixed berry crumble warm, either on its own or with a scoop of vanilla ice cream.

10. Enjoy the delightful combination of sweet berries and crunchy oat topping in this delicious dessert!

## Chia Seed Pudding with Berries

Ingredients:

- 1/4 cup chia seeds
- 1 cup unsweetened almond milk (or any other non-dairy milk)

- 2 tablespoons honey or maple syrup

- 1/2 teaspoon vanilla extract

- 1 cup mixed berries (strawberries, blueberries, raspberries)

- Fresh mint leaves for garnish

Instructions:

1. In a bowl, combine the chia seeds, almond milk, honey or maple syrup, and vanilla extract. Stir well to combine.

2. Let the mixture sit for 5 minutes, then stir again to prevent the chia seeds from clumping together.

3. Cover the bowl and refrigerate for at least 2 hours or overnight, allowing the chia seeds to absorb the liquid and create a pudding-like consistency.

4. When ready to serve, give the chia pudding a good stir to break up any clumps.

5. Divide the chia seed pudding into individual serving cups or bowls.

6. Top each portion with a generous amount of mixed berries.

7. Garnish with fresh mint leaves.

8. Serve chilled and enjoy this healthy and satisfying chia seed pudding with berries!

# Frozen Banana Bites with Dark Chocolate

Ingredients:

- 2 ripe bananas
- 1/4 cup dark chocolate chips
- 1 teaspoon coconut oil
- Chopped nuts or shredded coconut for coating (optional)

Instructions:

1. Peel the bananas and slice them into bite-sized pieces.
2. Place the banana slices on a baking sheet lined with parchment paper.
3. Insert a toothpick or small skewer into each banana slice, making it easier to handle.
4. Place the baking sheet in the freezer and freeze the banana slices for at least 1 hour or until completely frozen.

5. In a microwave-safe bowl, combine the dark chocolate chips and coconut oil.

6. Microwave in 30-second intervals, stirring in between, until the chocolate is melted and smooth.

7. Remove the frozen banana slices from the freezer.

8. Dip each banana slice into the melted chocolate, coating it completely.

9. If desired, roll the chocolate-coated banana slice in chopped nuts or shredded coconut.

10. Place the coated banana slices back on the parchment-lined baking sheet.

11. Return the baking sheet to the freezer and freeze for an additional 15-20 minutes or until the chocolate is set.

12. Once the chocolate is firm, remove the frozen banana bites from the freezer and transfer them to a container or zip-top bag for storage.

13. Enjoy these delightful frozen banana bites as a guilt-free treat!

# Lemon Blueberry Bars with Almond Crust

Ingredients:

- 1 1/2 cups almond flour
- 1/4 cup coconut flour
- 1/4 cup melted coconut oil
- 2 tablespoons honey or maple syrup
- 1 teaspoon vanilla extract
- 1/4 teaspoon salt
- 1 cup fresh blueberries
- Zest of 1 lemon
- Juice of 1 lemon
- 3 tablespoons honey or maple syrup
- 2 eggs

Instructions:

1. Preheat the oven to 350°F (175°C). Line a baking dish with parchment paper.
2. In a bowl, combine the almond flour, coconut flour, melted coconut oil, honey or maple syrup, vanilla extract, and salt. Mix well until a dough forms.

3. Press the dough evenly into the bottom of the lined baking dish to form the crust.

4. Bake the crust in the preheated oven for 10 minutes or until lightly golden.

5. While the crust is baking, prepare the lemon blueberry filling. In a separate bowl, whisk together the lemon zest, lemon juice, honey or maple syrup, and eggs until well combined.

6. Gently fold in the fresh blueberries.

7. Remove the crust from the oven and pour the lemon blueberry filling over the warm crust, spreading it out evenly.

8. Return the baking dish to the oven and bake for an additional 20-25 minutes or until the filling is set and the edges are golden brown.

9. Remove from the oven and let the lemon blueberry bars cool completely in the baking dish.

10. Once cooled, slice into bars and serve.

11. These lemon blueberry bars can be enjoyed at room temperature or chilled.

12. Indulge in the tangy-sweet flavors of these
    delightful lemon blueberry bars with an almond
    crust!


## Pumpkin Spice Energy Balls

Ingredients:

- 1 cup rolled oats
- 1/2 cup almond butter
- 1/4 cup pumpkin puree
- 1/4 cup honey or maple syrup
- 1/4 cup ground flaxseed
- 1/4 cup chopped walnuts
- 1 teaspoon pumpkin spice
- 1/2 teaspoon vanilla extract
- Pinch of salt
- Shredded coconut for rolling (optional)


Instructions:

1. In a bowl, combine the rolled oats, almond butter,
   pumpkin puree, honey or maple syrup, ground
   flaxseed, chopped walnuts, pumpkin spice, vanilla
   extract, and salt.

2. Stir well until all the ingredients are thoroughly combined.

3. Place the mixture in the refrigerator for 30 minutes to firm up.

4. After chilling, remove the mixture from the refrigerator and shape it into bite-sized balls using your hands.

5. If desired, roll the energy balls in shredded coconut for added texture and flavor.

6. Place the energy balls on a baking sheet lined with parchment paper.

7. Refrigerate the energy balls for at least 1 hour to allow them to set.

8. Once firm, transfer the pumpkin spice energy balls to a storage container and keep them refrigerated.

9. These energy balls make a perfect on-the-go snack or a quick pick-me-up during the day!

## Mango and Coconut Rice Pudding

Ingredients:

- 1 cup cooked brown rice
- 1 cup coconut milk

- 1 cup diced ripe mango
- 2 tablespoons honey or maple syrup
- 1/2 teaspoon vanilla extract
- Pinch of salt
- Toasted coconut flakes for garnish

Instructions:

1. In a saucepan, combine the cooked brown rice, coconut milk, diced mango, honey or maple syrup, vanilla extract, and salt.
2. Cook the mixture over medium heat, stirring frequently, until the coconut milk is absorbed and the pudding thickens to your desired consistency.
3. Remove the saucepan from the heat and let the rice pudding cool slightly.
4. Divide the rice pudding into serving bowls or glasses.
5. Garnish each portion with a sprinkle of toasted coconut flakes.
6. Serve the mango and coconut rice pudding warm or chilled.

7.  Enjoy the tropical flavors of this creamy and comforting dessert!

# Chapter 6: Smoothies

These smoothies are not only delicious but also packed with nutrients to support your well-being. Cheers to a refreshing and nutritious addition to your daily routine!

## Green Power Smoothie with Spinach and Kale

Ingredients:

- 1 cup fresh spinach leaves
- 1 cup chopped kale leaves
- 1 ripe banana
- 1 green apple, cored and chopped
- 1/2 cup cucumber, peeled and chopped
- 1/2 cup almond milk
- 1 tablespoon honey or maple syrup (optional)
- Ice cubes (optional)

Instructions:

1. In a blender, add the spinach, kale, banana, green apple, cucumber, and almond milk.

2. If desired, add honey or maple syrup for sweetness.

3. Blend on high speed until smooth and creamy.

4. If desired, add ice cubes and blend again until well incorporated.

5. Pour into a glass and enjoy this refreshing and nutrient-packed green smoothie.

## Berry Blast Smoothie with Greek Yogurt

Ingredients:

- 1 cup mixed berries (strawberries, blueberries, raspberries)
- 1/2 cup Greek yogurt
- 1/2 cup almond milk
- 1 tablespoon honey or agave syrup (optional)
- 1/2 teaspoon vanilla extract
- Ice cubes (optional)

Instructions:

1. In a blender, combine the mixed berries, Greek yogurt, almond milk, honey or agave syrup, and vanilla extract.

2.  Blend on high speed until the mixture is smooth and well combined.

3.  If desired, add ice cubes and blend again until the smoothie reaches the desired consistency.

4.  Pour into a glass and savor the delightful burst of berry flavors in this creamy and nutritious smoothie.

## Tropical Paradise Smoothie with Pineapple and Coconut

Ingredients:

- 1 cup frozen pineapple chunks
- 1/2 cup coconut milk
- 1/2 cup orange juice
- 1/4 cup plain Greek yogurt
- 1 tablespoon shredded coconut (optional)
- 1 teaspoon lime juice
- Ice cubes (optional)

Instructions:

1.  In a blender, add the frozen pineapple chunks, coconut milk, orange juice, Greek yogurt, shredded coconut (if using), and lime juice.

2. Blend on high speed until all the ingredients are thoroughly mixed and the smoothie is creamy.

3. If desired, add ice cubes and blend again until the smoothie reaches the desired consistency.

4. Pour into a glass and transport yourself to a tropical paradise with this refreshing and luscious smoothie.

## Chocolate Peanut Butter Banana Smoothie

Ingredients:

- 1 ripe banana
- 1 tablespoon unsweetened cocoa powder
- 2 tablespoons peanut butter
- 1 cup almond milk
- 1 tablespoon honey or maple syrup (optional)
- Ice cubes (optional)

Instructions:

1. In a blender, combine the ripe banana, cocoa powder, peanut butter, almond milk, and honey or maple syrup (if desired).

2. Blend on high speed until the mixture is smooth and creamy.

3. If desired, add ice cubes and blend again until the smoothie is chilled and well blended.

4. Pour into a glass and indulge in the delectable combination of chocolate, peanut butter, and banana in this satisfying smoothie.

## Spinach and Mango Smoothie with Almond Milk

Ingredients:

- 1 cup fresh spinach leaves
- 1 cup chopped ripe mango
- 1/2 cup almond milk
- 1/2 cup plain Greek yogurt
- 1 tablespoon honey or agave syrup (optional)
- Ice cubes (optional)

Instructions:

1. In a blender, add the spinach leaves, chopped mango, almond milk, Greek yogurt, and honey or agave syrup (if desired).

2. Blend on high speed until all the ingredients are well incorporated and the smoothie is creamy.

3. If desired, add ice cubes and blend again until the smoothie is chilled and has a smooth consistency.

4. Pour into a glass and enjoy the vibrant flavors and health benefits of spinach and mango in this invigorating smoothie.

## Antioxidant-Rich Blueberry Smoothie

Ingredients:

- 1 cup blueberries
- 1/2 cup almond milk
- 1/2 cup plain Greek yogurt
- 1 tablespoon chia seeds
- 1 tablespoon honey or agave syrup (optional)
- Ice cubes (optional)

Instructions:

1. In a blender, combine the blueberries, almond milk, Greek yogurt, chia seeds, and honey or agave syrup (if desired).

2.  Blend on high speed until the mixture is smooth and creamy.

3.  If desired, add ice cubes and blend again until the smoothie is chilled and well blended.

4.  Pour into a glass and relish the antioxidant-rich goodness of blueberries in this delightful smoothie.

## Peach and Ginger Smoothie with Flaxseed

Ingredients:

- 1 cup chopped ripe peaches
- 1/2 cup almond milk
- 1/2 cup plain Greek yogurt
- 1 tablespoon flaxseed meal
- 1 teaspoon grated fresh ginger
- 1 tablespoon honey or agave syrup (optional)
- Ice cubes (optional)

Instructions:

1.  In a blender, add the chopped peaches, almond milk, Greek yogurt, flaxseed meal, grated ginger, and honey or agave syrup (if desired).

2.  Blend on high speed until all the ingredients are
    thoroughly combined and the smoothie is creamy.

3.  If desired, add ice cubes and blend again until the
    smoothie is chilled and has a smooth texture.

4.  Pour into a glass and savor the delightful
    combination of sweet peaches and zingy ginger in
    this invigorating smoothie.

## Raspberry and Almond Butter Smoothie

Ingredients:

- 1 cup raspberries
- 2 tablespoons almond butter
- 1/2 cup almond milk
- 1/2 cup plain Greek yogurt
- 1 tablespoon honey or agave syrup (optional)
- Ice cubes (optional)

Instructions:

1.  In a blender, combine the raspberries, almond
    butter, almond milk, Greek yogurt, and honey or
    agave syrup (if desired).

2. Blend on high speed until the mixture is smooth and creamy.

3. If desired, add ice cubes and blend again until the smoothie is chilled and well blended.

4. Pour into a glass and enjoy the delightful combination of tangy raspberries and nutty almond butter in this satisfying smoothie.

## Pineapple and Cucumber Smoothie with Mint

Ingredients:

- 1 cup frozen pineapple chunks
- 1/2 cup cucumber, peeled and chopped
- 1/2 cup coconut water
- 1 tablespoon lime juice
- 1 tablespoon fresh mint leaves
- 1 tablespoon honey or agave syrup (optional)
- Ice cubes (optional)

Instructions:

1.  In a blender, add the frozen pineapple chunks, cucumber, coconut water, lime juice, mint leaves, and honey or agave syrup (if desired).
2.  Blend on high speed until all the ingredients are well combined and the smoothie is creamy.
3.  If desired, add ice cubes and blend again until the smoothie is chilled and has a smooth texture.
4.  Pour into a glass and enjoy the refreshing and hydrating flavors of pineapple, cucumber, and mint in this revitalizing smoothie.

## Coffee and Banana Smoothie with Oatmeal

Ingredients:

- 1 ripe banana
- 1/2 cup brewed coffee, cooled
- 1/2 cup almond milk
- 1/4 cup rolled oats
- 1 tablespoon almond butter
- 1 tablespoon honey or maple syrup (optional)
- Ice cubes (optional)

Instructions:

1. In a blender, combine the ripe banana, brewed coffee, almond milk, rolled oats, almond butter, and honey or maple syrup (if desired).

2. Blend on high speed until the mixture is smooth and creamy.

3. If desired, add ice cubes and blend again until the smoothie is chilled and well blended.

4. Pour into a glass and enjoy the energizing combination of coffee, banana, and oats in this satisfying smoothie.

# CONCLUSION

Before bidding farewell, let us take a moment to recap the key principles of heart-healthy diabetic cooking that we have emphasized throughout this cookbook. These principles serve as a foundation for creating meals that are both beneficial for your heart and suitable for diabetes management.

First and foremost, we have emphasized the importance of a balanced and varied diet. A diverse range of nutrients, vitamins, and minerals is essential for overall health and well-being. Incorporating a wide array of fruits, vegetables, whole grains, lean proteins, and healthy fats into your meals is crucial for maintaining a healthy heart and stable blood sugar levels.

Additionally, we have stressed the significance of portion control. While the quality of ingredients matters, the quantity we consume is equally important. By monitoring portion sizes and practicing mindful eating, we can prevent overeating and maintain a healthy weight, which is crucial for managing diabetes and reducing the risk of heart-related complications.

Moreover, we have highlighted the significance of choosing low-glycemic index foods. These are foods that have a minimal impact on blood sugar levels, making them suitable for individuals with diabetes. By opting for whole grains, legumes, non-starchy vegetables, and lean proteins, we can help stabilize blood glucose levels and promote better glycemic control.

**Long-Term Strategies for Maintaining a Healthy Lifestyle**

Beyond the recipes and meal plans provided in this cookbook, it is essential to consider long-term strategies for maintaining a healthy lifestyle. Here are a few additional tips to help you on your journey towards heart-healthy diabetic living:

- Regular Physical Activity: Incorporate regular exercise into your routine, as it plays a crucial role in managing diabetes and promoting cardiovascular health. Engage in activities you enjoy, such as walking, swimming, cycling, or dancing.

- Stress Management: Chronic stress can negatively impact both diabetes and heart health. Find healthy outlets to manage stress, such as meditation, yoga, deep breathing exercises, or engaging in hobbies that bring you joy.

- Regular Check-ups: Schedule regular check-ups with your healthcare provider to monitor your blood sugar levels, blood pressure, cholesterol, and overall health. These routine visits allow for early detection and management of any potential health issues.

- Continuous Learning: Stay informed about the latest research, guidelines, and advancements in diabetes and heart health management. Education empowers you to make informed decisions about your health and well-being.